Healing Heart Diseases: A Nutrition Based Approach For

A Healthy Heart

DISCLAIMER

The information contained in this resource is general in nature and for informative purposes only.

The Author assumes no responsibility whatsoever, under any circumstances, for any actions taken as a result of the information contained herein.

You are required to seek professional help if needed.

Before this document is duplicated or reproduced

in any manner, the publisher's consent must be

gained. Therefore, the contents within can neither

be stored electronically, transferred, nor kept in a

database.

Neither in Part nor full can the document be

copied, scanned, faxed, or retained without

approval from the publisher or creator.

Copyright © by Leo Chambers 2024. All rights

reserved

Preface

The human heart, a tireless pump silently working away, is the very essence of life. Yet, for many, this vital organ becomes a source of concern. Heart disease, encompassing a variety of conditions, remains a leading cause of illness and death worldwide.

This book is intended to be your companion on the journey towards understanding heart disease. Whether you are a patient seeking knowledge, a healthcare professional looking for a refresher, or simply someone concerned about your heart health, this book offers a clear and comprehensive guide.

Within these pages, we will delve into the various forms of heart disease, exploring their causes, symptoms, and available treatments. We will discuss the latest advancements in medical technology and explore preventative measures you can take to safeguard your heart's health.

Most importantly, this book empowers you with knowledge. With a deeper understanding of heart disease, you can make informed decisions about your health and work collaboratively with your doctor to achieve the best possible outcome. This journey may seem daunting, but fear not. We will navigate it together, one informative chapter at a time.

Leo Chambers

Contents

Introduction:

A Journey to Heart Health

Understanding Heart Disease

In the quiet of a hospital room, amidst beeping monitors and hushed conversations, Sarah sat by her father's bedside. The diagnosis had come like a thunderclap—coronary artery disease, a silent intruder that had crept into her father's life, threatening to steal precious moments, laughter, and shared memories.

Heart disease, she realized, was not just a medical condition; it was a journey—a journey of challenges, uncertainties, and choices that would redefine their family's path ahead. Sarah delved into the depths of understanding heart disease, unraveling its complexities, causes, and impact on millions of lives worldwide.

Heart disease, she learned, encompasses a spectrum of conditions—from coronary artery disease and heart attacks to heart failure, arrhythmias, and congenital heart defects. It's a multifaceted landscape, shaped by genetics, lifestyle factors, environmental influences, and medical advancements.

Importance of Nutrition in Heart Health

As Sarah embarked on her quest for knowledge, she encountered a recurring theme—a theme that resonated through medical journals, research studies, and conversations with healthcare experts: the pivotal role of nutrition in heart health.

Nutrition, she discovered, was not just about calorie counts or dietary fads; it was about nourishing the body, protecting the heart, and fostering a foundation of wellness. The foods we consume, Sarah realized, could either fuel inflammation, cholesterol buildup, and cardiovascular risks, or they could become potent allies in preventing and reversing heart disease.

Overview of Recent Advancements

In the realm of heart health, progress is not stagnant—it's a dynamic landscape shaped by relentless innovation, breakthrough discoveries, and cutting-edge advancements. Sarah delved into the world of recent advancements, uncovering a treasure trove of scientific insights, technological innovations, and novel approaches to cardiac care.

From genetic testing and precision medicine to personalized nutrition plans and targeted therapies, the landscape of heart disease management was evolving. Sarah marveled at the strides made in early detection, minimally invasive procedures, and holistic approaches that embraced the interconnectedness of mind, body, and heart.

This introduction sets the stage for a captivating journey—a journey of understanding, empowerment, and transformation in the realm of heart health. As Sarah navigates the complexities of heart disease and the transformative power of nutrition-based cures and recent advancements, she invites readers to embark on a quest for heart health—a quest fueled by knowledge, resilience, and hope.

Chapter 1

Foundations of Heart Health

1. Life systems and Capability of the Heart

Disclosing the Heart's Secrets

The heart — a wonder of organic designing, an image of life's cadence, and a stalwart that supports our reality. To comprehend coronary illness and its avoidance, we should initially disentangle the many-sided life structures and dynamic capability of this crucial organ.

The heart, settled defensively inside the chest cavity, is a solid siphon that indefatigably courses blood all through the body. Its chambers — four altogether — contain the right chamber, right ventricle, left chamber, and left ventricle, each assuming an exceptional part in the dissemination of oxygen-rich blood and oxygen-exhausted blood.

As we dive further into the heart's chambers, valves, supply routes, and veins, we uncover the perfect dance of systole and diastole — the musical constrictions and relaxations that move blood stream, keep up with pulse, and sustain each cell, tissue, and organ with oxygen and supplements.

The Circulatory Ensemble

Picture the heart as the director of a fantastic ensemble — the circulatory framework. Supply routes, similar to the superb strings, divert oxygen-rich blood from the heart to the body's tissues and organs. Veins, similar to the agreeable woodwinds, get oxygen-drained blood once again to the heart for reestablishment.

The coronary conduits, fragile branches that embrace the heart like defensive ringlets, supply oxygen and supplements to the heart muscle itself, guaranteeing its consistent essentialness and capability. Any disturbance in this ensemble — be it atherosclerosis, plaque development, or blood vessel blockages — can prompt coronary illness, upsetting the agreeable progression of life.

The Electrical Symphony

Past its mechanical ability, the heart houses a perplexing electrical framework — the cardiovascular conduction framework. Like talented performers in a symphony, specific cells create electrical driving forces that coordinate pulses, beat, and timing. The sinoatrial (SA) hub, the heart's regular pacemaker, organizes every heartbeat with accuracy, guaranteeing a synchronized ensemble of compressions.

Understanding the heart's life systems and capability lays the preparation for appreciating how coronary illness can upset this ensemble, prompting conditions, for example, coronary course infection, coronary episodes, arrhythmias, cardiovascular breakdown, and innate deformities.

2. Normal Types and Reasons for Coronary illness

Exposing the Causes of Coronary illness

Coronary illness is definitely not a solitary substance; it includes a range of conditions, each with its interesting qualities, causes, and suggestions for heart wellbeing. As we explore this scene, we experience normal kinds of coronary illness and their basic causes:

  - Coronary Vein Infection (computer aided design): The main source of coronary illness, computer aided design emerges from the slow development of plaque — a combination of cholesterol, greasy stores, and cell garbage — inside the coronary conduits. This limiting of the supply routes confines blood stream to the heart muscle, prompting angina (chest pain), respiratory failures, and myocardial areas of localized necrosis.

  - Cardiovascular failures (Myocardial Areas of dead tissue): A coronary failure happens when a coronary course turns out to be unexpectedly impeded, denying a part of the heart muscle of oxygen and supplements. The subsequent harm can be perilous, requiring brief clinical mediation to reestablish blood stream and forestall further difficulties.

- Arrhythmias: Sporadic heart rhythms, or arrhythmias, can disturb the heart's electrical motivations, prompting palpitations, wooziness, swooning, and possibly perilous difficulties like ventricular fibrillation or unexpected heart failure.

- Cardiovascular breakdown: In opposition to its name, cardiovascular breakdown doesn't suggest a discontinuance of heart capability yet rather a decreased capacity of the heart to effectively siphon blood. Reasons for cardiovascular breakdown include basic circumstances like hypertension, diabetes, coronary supply route infection, valvular problems, and cardiomyopathies.

- Innate Heart Deformities: A few people are brought into the world with primary irregularities in the heart, known as inherent heart surrenders. These imperfections can go from straightforward physical varieties to complex deformities that influence heart capability and flow.

- Valvular Coronary illness: Brokenness or anomalies in the heart valves — structures that manage blood stream inside the heart — can prompt valvular coronary illness. Conditions like valve stenosis (limiting) or disgorging (spillage) can strain the heart and weaken its proficiency.

Understanding the types and reasons for coronary illness enlightens the multifactorial idea of cardiovascular wellbeing, affected by hereditary qualities, lifestyle factors, natural openings, age, orientation, and basic ailments.

3. Risk Variables and Avoidance Methodologies

Disclosing the Embroidery of Hazard

Coronary illness is frequently named the "quiet executioner" for its guileful nature, unobtrusively advancing over years or a very long time prior to appearing as side effects or complexities. As we peer into the woven artwork of hazard factors, we experience both modifiable and non-modifiable components that impact heart wellbeing:

- Non-Modifiable Risk Elements:

- Hereditary qualities and Family Ancestry: Acquired characteristics and family background of coronary illness can expand helplessness to cardiovascular circumstances.

- Age and Orientation: Propelling age and male orientation are related with expanded risk, in spite of the fact that coronary illness influences people of any age and sexes.

- Identity: Certain ethnic gatherings, like African Americans, Hispanics, and Local Americans, may have a higher inclination to coronary illness.

- Modifiable Risk Variables:

- Hypertension (Hypertension): Raised pulse strains the heart and conduits, adding to atherosclerosis and cardiovascular inconveniences.

- Dyslipidemia (Elevated Cholesterol): Uneven characters in cholesterol levels, especially raised LDL cholesterol ("awful" cholesterol) and low HDL cholesterol ("great" cholesterol), can advance plaque arrangement and conduit limiting.

- Diabetes Mellitus: Diabetes, particularly inadequately controlled diabetes, speeds up atherosclerosis, increments cardiovascular dangers, and disables heart capability.

- Stoutness and Inactive Way of life: Overabundance body weight, especially stomach heftiness, and a stationary way of life are connected to irritation, insulin opposition, hypertension, dyslipidemia, and coronary illness.

- Smoking and Tobacco Use: Cigarette smoking and tobacco use harm veins and promote atherosclerosis as well as add to arrhythmias, blood thickening, and coronary failures.

- Lack of Eating regimen: Diets high in soaked fats, trans fats, cholesterol, sodium, and refined sugars can fuel irritation, raise circulatory strain, deteriorate lipid profiles, and increase cardiovascular dangers.

- Actual Latency: Absence of customary active work debilitates the heart, impedes dissemination, advances weight gain, worsens metabolic lopsided characteristics, and adds to coronary illness.

- Stress and Psychological well-being: Ongoing pressure, tension, misery, and annoying intense subject matters can strain the heart, raise pulse, modify heart rhythms, and affect general cardiovascular wellbeing.

- Liquor and Substance Misuse: Exorbitant liquor utilization, illegal medication use, and substance misuse can harm the heart muscle, disturb heart rhythms, add to hypertension, and increase the risk of coronary illness.

- Lack of Quality Rest: Insufficient rest, rest issues, and rest unsettling influences can debilitate heart capability, disturb circadian rhythms, advance irritation, and raise cardiovascular dangers.

By understanding these risk factors — both modifiable and non-modifiable — we gain knowledge into the complicated transaction of hereditary inclination, way of life decisions, ecological impacts, and by and large heart wellbeing.

Engaging Counteraction Procedures

Furnished with information, people can leave on a proactive journey of counteraction, embracing proof based procedures to defend heart wellbeing, relieve chances, and promote by and large wellbeing. These techniques include:

  - **Good dieting Propensities**: Embracing a heart-sound eating routine wealthy in organic products, vegetables, entire grains, lean proteins, solid fats (like omega-3 unsaturated fats), and fiber. Restricting intake of soaked fats, trans fats, cholesterol, sodium, and added sugars is critical to diminishing cardiovascular dangers.

  - **Customary Actual work**: Integrating standard activity and actual work into everyday schedules, holding back nothing 150 minutes of moderate-force oxygen consuming movement or 75 minutes of fiery power action each week, alongside muscle-reinforcing exercises on at least two days of the week.

- **Keeping a Sound Weight**: Accomplishing and keeping a solid body weight through a blend of adjusted nourishment, normal active work, segment control, careful eating, and way of life changes.

- **Overseeing Pulse**: Checking circulatory strain routinely, embracing way of life adjustments (like dietary changes, actual work, stress management and lessening sodium intake), and following clinical suggestions for hypertension management.

- **Improving Cholesterol Levels**: Observing lipid profiles (counting LDL cholesterol, HDL cholesterol, and fatty oils), executing dietary alterations (like diminishing immersed fats, trans fats, and cholesterol admission), and taking into account medicine treatment if essential.

- **Overseeing Diabetes and Glucose Levels**: Controlling blood glucose levels through smart dieting, normal actual work, medicine adherence (whenever recommended), glucose checking, and diabetes the board methodologies custom fitted to individual necessities.

- **Tobacco Cessation:** Stopping smoking, keeping away from openness to handed-down cigarette smoke, and looking for help, advising, and smoking end projects to defeat nicotine habit and decrease cardiovascular dangers.

- **Stress Management**: Implementing stress-reducing techniques, relaxation therapies, mindfulness practices, meditation, yoga, counseling, and seeking support networks to manage stress, anxiety, and emotional well-being.

- **Quality Sleep**: Prioritizing quality sleep, establishing consistent sleep patterns, creating a sleep-friendly environment, addressing sleep disorders or disturbances, and practicing good sleep hygiene for restorative rest and optimal cardiovascular health.

- **Limiting Alcohol and Substance Use**: Moderating alcohol consumption, avoiding excessive drinking, abstaining from illicit drugs and substance abuse, and seeking assistance or treatment for addiction or dependency issues.

By adopting these preventive strategies, individuals can empower themselves to take control of their heart health, reduce cardiovascular risks, and enhance overall well-being. Prevention is not merely a concept—it's a proactive choice, a commitment to nurturing a healthy heart and a fulfilling life.

This detailed exploration of the foundations of heart health provides a comprehensive understanding of the heart's anatomy, common types and causes of heart disease, and effective prevention strategies. Armed with knowledge, individuals can embark on a transformative journey towards optimal heart health, embracing lifestyle modifications, healthy habits, and proactive measures to safeguard their cardiovascular well-being.

Chapter 2

Nutrition-Based Approach

The Role of Nutrition in Heart Disease

Fueling Heart Health

Nutrition is not merely about sustenance—it's a powerful tool for nurturing heart health, combating inflammation, optimizing cholesterol levels, managing blood pressure, supporting overall cardiovascular function, and reducing the risk of heart disease.

Key Nutrients for Heart Health

 - **Omega-3 Fatty Acids:** Found in fatty fish (such as salmon, mackerel, sardines), flaxseeds, chia seeds, walnuts, and algae-based supplements, omega-3 fatty acids are renowned for their anti-inflammatory properties, cardiovascular benefits, and potential to lower triglyceride levels, reduce arrhythmias, and support heart function.

 - **Fiber:** Abundant in fruits, vegetables, whole grains, legumes, nuts, and seeds, dietary fiber plays a crucial role in cholesterol management, blood sugar regulation, weight management, digestive health, and reducing cardiovascular risks such as hypertension and atherosclerosis.

- **Antioxidants**: Found in colorful fruits, vegetables, berries, nuts, seeds, and dark chocolate, antioxidants (such as vitamins C and E, beta-carotene, flavonoids, and polyphenols) combat oxidative stress, reduce inflammation, protect against cellular damage, and promote heart health.

- **Plant Sterols and Stanols:** Naturally occurring compounds in plant-based foods (like fruits, vegetables, whole grains, nuts, and seeds) or added to fortified products, plant sterols and stanols help lower LDL cholesterol levels, support cholesterol balance, and reduce cardiovascular risks.

- **Potassium and Magnesium**: Abundant in fruits, vegetables, legumes, nuts, seeds, and whole grains, potassium and magnesium play vital roles in blood pressure regulation, electrolyte balance, heart rhythm stability, and cardiovascular health.

- **Healthy Fats**: Opt for heart-healthy fats, such as monounsaturated fats (found in olive oil, avocados, nuts, and seeds) and polyunsaturated fats (including omega-3 and omega-6 fatty acids), while limiting saturated fats and avoiding trans fats to promote optimal lipid profiles and heart health.

 - **Low Glycemic Index Foods**: Choosing low glycemic index (GI) foods—such as whole grains, legumes, non-starchy vegetables, and fruits with a moderate glycemic load—can help manage blood sugar levels, reduce insulin resistance, and lower the risk of diabetes-related heart complications.

. Heart-Healthy Diet Guidelines

Crafting a Nutrient-Dense Plate

Building upon the foundation of key nutrients, a heart-healthy diet emphasizes whole, minimally processed foods, plant-based options, lean proteins, healthy fats, and mindful eating practices. Let's explore the essential components of a heart-healthy diet:

 - **Fruits and Vegetables**: Aim for a rainbow of colors, incorporating a variety of fruits and vegetables rich in vitamins, minerals, antioxidants, fiber, and phytonutrients. Include leafy greens, berries, citrus fruits, cruciferous vegetables, tomatoes, carrots, and peppers in your daily meals.

- **Whole Grains**: Opt for whole grains such as brown rice, quinoa, barley, oats, whole wheat, bulgur, and farro over refined grains. Whole grains offer fiber, B vitamins, minerals, and sustained energy without the rapid blood sugar spikes associated with refined grains.

- **Legumes and Pulses:** Include beans, lentils, chickpeas, peas, and soy products in your diet for plant-based protein, fiber, complex carbohydrates, and beneficial nutrients that promote heart health, satiety, and blood sugar control.

- **Healthy Fats**: Incorporate sources of healthy fats, such as avocados, olives, olive oil, nuts (like almonds, walnuts, pistachios), seeds (such as chia, flaxseeds, hemp seeds), and fatty fish (like salmon, mackerel, trout), into your meals to support heart function, inflammation reduction, and cholesterol balance.

- **Lean Proteins:** Choose lean protein sources such as poultry (skinless chicken, turkey), fish, seafood, tofu, tempeh, legumes, low-fat dairy (such as Greek yogurt, cottage cheese), and eggs to meet your protein needs while minimizing saturated fat intake.

   - **Dairy and Alternatives:** Opt for low-fat or fat-free dairy products (like milk, yogurt, cheese) or plant-based alternatives (such as almond milk, soy milk, coconut yogurt) to ensure adequate calcium, vitamin D, and protein intake while managing saturated fat content.

   - **Limit Sodium and Added Sugars:** Reduce sodium intake by choosing low-sodium or no-added-salt options, seasoning foods with herbs, spices, citrus, and vinegar instead of salt, and reading labels for hidden sodium sources. Minimize added sugars by selecting whole foods, reducing sugary beverages

Chapter 3

Nutrition-Based Interventions

Plant-Based Diet for Heart Disease Prevention and Reversal

The Power of Plants

Embracing a plant-based diet can be a transformative step in preventing and reversing heart disease. This dietary approach focuses on whole plant foods while minimizing or excluding animal products and processed foods high in saturated fats, cholesterol, and sodium.

- Benefits of a Plant-Based Diet:

- Heart Health: Plant-based diets are rich in fiber, antioxidants, vitamins, minerals, and phytonutrients that promote cardiovascular health, reduce inflammation, lower cholesterol levels, improve blood pressure, and support overall heart function.

- Weight Management: Plant-based diets tend to be lower in calories, saturated fats, and processed sugars, making them conducive to weight management, reducing body mass index (BMI), and lowering the risk of obesity-related heart complications.

- Blood Sugar Control: Plant-based diets can improve insulin sensitivity, regulate blood sugar levels, reduce the risk of type 2 diabetes, and mitigate diabetes-related cardiovascular risks.

- Gut Health: The abundance of fiber and prebiotics in plant-based foods nourishes beneficial gut bacteria, supports digestive health, enhances nutrient absorption, and may reduce systemic inflammation linked to heart disease.

- Anti-Inflammatory Effects: Plant-based diets are associated with lower levels of inflammatory markers, such as C-reactive protein (CRP), interleukin-6 (IL-6), and tumor necrosis factor-alpha (TNF-alpha), which play a role in cardiovascular disease progression.

- Blood Lipid Improvement: Consuming plant-based foods can lead to favorable changes in lipid profiles, including reductions in LDL cholesterol ("bad" cholesterol), triglycerides, and total cholesterol levels, while increasing HDL cholesterol ("good" cholesterol") levels.

- Blood Pressure Reduction: The potassium-rich and sodium-limited nature of plant-based diets contributes to lower blood pressure, improved vascular health, and reduced hypertension risks.

- **Components of a Plant-Based Diet:**

  - Whole Grains: Incorporate whole grains like quinoa, brown rice, oats, barley, bulgur, whole wheat, and farro for fiber, complex carbohydrates, vitamins, minerals, and sustained energy.

  - Fruits and Vegetables: Aim for a colorful array of fruits and vegetables, including leafy greens, berries, citrus fruits, cruciferous vegetables, tomatoes, carrots, peppers, and more, to provide antioxidants, vitamins, minerals, and phytonutrients.

  - Legumes and Pulses: Include beans, lentils, chickpeas, peas, soy products, and legume-based foods for plant-based protein, fiber, iron, folate, and beneficial nutrients.

  - Nuts and Seeds: Enjoy moderate portions of nuts (like almonds, walnuts, pistachios, cashews) and seeds (such as chia, flaxseeds, hemp seeds, pumpkin seeds) for healthy fats, protein, fiber, vitamins, minerals, and omega-3 fatty acids.

- Plant-Based Proteins: Incorporate tofu, tempeh, edamame, seitan, and plant-based protein sources into meals for variety, protein diversity, and meat-free alternatives.

- Healthy Fats: Include sources of healthy fats like avocados, olives, olive oil, and plant-based oils in moderation to support heart health, inflammation reduction, and nutrient absorption.

- Herbs and Spices: Use herbs, spices, seasonings, and natural flavor enhancers (like garlic, ginger, turmeric, cinnamon, cumin, paprika) to add depth, aroma, and taste to plant-based dishes without excess salt or added sugars.

Transitioning to a Plant-Based Lifestyle

Transitioning to a plant-based diet can be a gradual and sustainable process, starting with small changes, experimenting with new recipes, exploring plant-based alternatives, and seeking guidance from healthcare professionals or registered dietitians. Focus on diversity, balance, nutrient adequacy, and enjoyment in your plant-based journey, recognizing the multitude of health benefits it offers for heart disease prevention and management.

Mediterranean Diet and Heart Health

Savoring the Mediterranean Way

The Mediterranean diet—a culinary treasure trove inspired by the traditional dietary patterns of Mediterranean countries like Greece, Italy, Spain, and Southern France—has garnered global recognition for its heart-healthy benefits, culinary delights, and cultural richness.

- **Principles of the Mediterranean Diet:**

- Abundance of Plant Foods: Emphasizes fruits, vegetables, legumes, nuts, seeds, whole grains, herbs, and spices as foundational elements, providing fiber, antioxidants, vitamins, minerals, and phytonutrients.

- Olive Oil as Primary Fat Source: Utilizes extra virgin olive oil as the primary source of fat, rich in monounsaturated fats, polyphenols, and antioxidants that promote heart health, inflammation reduction, and lipid balance.

- Moderate Fish and Poultry Consumption: Includes moderate consumption of fish (especially fatty fish like salmon, sardines, mackerel) and poultry (like chicken, turkey) as protein sources, offering omega-3 fatty acids, lean protein, and essential nutrients.

- Limited Red Meat and Dairy: Restricts red meat consumption (such as beef, pork, lamb) to occasional or smaller portions and emphasizes lean protein sources. Moderates dairy intake, with preference for low-fat or fermented dairy products (like yogurt, cheese).

- Emphasis on Flavorful Foods: Enhances culinary creations with herbs, spices, garlic, onions, citrus, vinegar, and natural flavor enhancers to add depth, aroma, and taste without excess salt, sugar, or processed ingredients.

- Enjoyment of Wine in Moderation: Permits moderate consumption of red wine (in the context of cultural traditions and individual preferences) for its potential cardiovascular benefits, antioxidants (like resveratrol), and social enjoyment.

- Mindful Eating and Social Engagement: Encourages mindful eating practices, savoring meals, enjoying shared meals with family and friends, fostering social connections, and promoting holistic well-being beyond nutritional considerations.

- Heart-Healthy Benefits of the Mediterranean Diet:

- Cardiovascular Protection: The Mediterranean diet's emphasis on plant foods, healthy fats (like olive oil and omega-3-rich fish), lean proteins, and moderate alcohol intake is associated with reduced cardiovascular risks, lower incidence of heart disease, and improved heart health markers.

- Anti-Inflammatory Effects: The abundance of antioxidants, polyphenols, and omega-3 fatty acids in Mediterranean foods contributes to inflammation reduction and supports optimal immune function, cellular health, and vascular integrity, thereby reducing the risk of inflammatory-driven heart conditions.

- Cholesterol and Lipid Management: The Mediterranean diet's focus on monounsaturated fats (from olive oil), omega-3 fatty acids (from fish), and fiber-rich foods (like fruits, vegetables, and whole grains) promotes favorable lipid profiles, lowers LDL cholesterol levels, raises HDL cholesterol levels, and supports overall lipid balance.

   - **Blood Pressure Regulation**: The combination of potassium-rich foods (such as leafy greens, bananas, legumes) and sodium moderation in the Mediterranean diet contributes to lower blood pressure, improved vascular tone, enhanced endothelial function, and reduced hypertension risks.

   - **Blood Sugar Control**: The Mediterranean diet's emphasis on whole, unprocessed foods, complex carbohydrates, fiber, and healthy fats promotes stable blood sugar levels, insulin sensitivity, glycemic control, and reduced diabetes-related cardiovascular complication management.

Weight Management: The Mediterranean diet's nutrient-dense, plant-centric approach, along with portion control, mindful eating, and enjoyment of satiating foods, supports healthy weight management, reduces abdominal adiposity, and lowers obesity-related heart risks.

Adopting the Mediterranean Lifestyle

Transitioning to a Mediterranean-inspired lifestyle involves embracing culinary diversity, seasonal ingredients, mindful eating practices, social engagement, and enjoyment of wholesome, flavorful foods. Incorporate these key elements into your daily routine to experience the heart-healthy benefits and vibrant flavors of the Mediterranean diet.

DASH Diet for Blood Pressure Management

Balancing Blood Pressure with DASH

The Dietary Approaches to Stop Hypertension (DASH) diet is a science-backed dietary pattern renowned for its effectiveness in lowering blood pressure, promoting heart health, and reducing cardiovascular risks, making it a valuable tool in managing hypertension and supporting overall cardiovascular well-being.

- Core Principles of the DASH Diet:

- Abundance of Fruits and Vegetables: Emphasizes a variety of colorful fruits, vegetables, legumes, and whole grains rich in potassium, magnesium, fiber, antioxidants, and phytonutrients that support blood pressure regulation, vascular health, and heart function.

- Moderation of Sodium: Limits sodium intake to 2,300 milligrams per day (or even lower, to 1,500 milligrams) by choosing low-sodium or no-added-salt options, reducing processed and packaged foods, using herbs, spices, and natural flavorings, and reading labels for hidden sodium sources.

- Lean Protein Sources: Incorporates lean proteins like poultry, fish, beans, lentils, tofu, and low-fat dairy products as protein sources, reducing saturated fats and cholesterol while providing essential nutrients.

- Whole Grains and Fiber: Prioritizes whole grains (such as brown rice, whole wheat, oats, quinoa, barley) and fiber-rich foods for sustained energy, digestive health, blood sugar control, and satiety, while avoiding refined grains and added sugars.

- Healthy Fats: Includes sources of healthy fats like nuts, seeds, avocados, olive oil, and fatty fish (like salmon, trout) to provide monounsaturated fats, omega-3 fatty acids, and antioxidant compounds that support heart health and inflammation reduction.

- Limited Red Meat and Sweets: Reduces consumption of red meats, processed meats, sugary beverages, desserts, and high-fat snacks to minimize saturated fats, excess calories, added sugars, and unhealthy food choices.

-Benefits of the DASH Diet for Heart Health:

- Blood Pressure Reduction: The DASH diet's emphasis on potassium-rich foods, low sodium intake, balanced nutrients, and heart-healthy choices contributes to lower blood pressure, improved vascular tone, reduced hypertension risks, and enhanced cardiovascular function.

- Lipid and Cholesterol Improvement: Adopting the DASH diet can lead to favorable changes in lipid profiles, including reductions in LDL cholesterol levels, triglycerides, and total cholesterol, while increasing HDL cholesterol levels, supporting lipid balance, and reducing cardiovascular risks.

- Weight Management: The nutrient-dense, fiber-rich nature of the DASH diet promotes satiety, regulates appetite, supports weight loss or weight maintenance, and reduces obesity-related heart complications.

- Diabetes and Blood Sugar Control: The DASH diet's focus on whole, unprocessed foods, complex carbohydrates, fiber, and nutrient-rich choices can help stabilize blood sugar levels, improve insulin sensitivity, and reduce the risk of diabetes-related cardiovascular issues.

Implementing the DASH Lifestyle

Adopting the DASH lifestyle involves strategic meal planning, grocery shopping, label reading, portion control, mindful eating, and regular monitoring of blood pressure and dietary choices. Collaborate with healthcare professionals, registered dietitians, and lifestyle coaches to customize the DASH diet to your unique needs, preferences, and health goals for optimal blood pressure management and heart health.

Nutrition for Diabetes Management and Heart Health

Navigating Diabetes and Heart Disease

Diabetes and heart disease often intersect, with diabetes acting as a significant risk factor for cardiovascular complications. Nutrition plays a pivotal role in diabetes management, blood sugar control, insulin sensitivity, and mitigating diabetes-related heart risks, making dietary interventions a cornerstone of comprehensive care.

- **Impact of Diabetes on Heart Health:**

- Cardiovascular Risks: Diabetes is associated with increased cardiovascular risks, including coronary artery disease, myocardial infarction, stroke, peripheral artery disease, heart failure, and microvascular complications that affect the heart, blood vessels, and circulation.

- Metabolic Imbalances: Diabetes can lead to metabolic imbalances, insulin resistance, hyperglycemia, dyslipidemia, hypertension, inflammation, oxidative stress, endothelial dysfunction, and abnormal lipid profiles, contributing to heart disease development and progression.

- Heart-Related Complications: Diabetes-related heart complications may include atherosclerosis, coronary artery disease, myocardial ischemia, heart attacks, arrhythmias, heart failure, diabetic cardiomyopathy, and increased cardiovascular mortality rates.

- **Nutritional Strategies for Diabetes and Heart Health:**

- Blood Sugar Management: Focus on carbohydrate counting, glycemic index/load awareness, portion control, meal timing, balanced meals/snacks, blood glucose monitoring, insulin/oral medication adherence, and personalized nutrition plans to manage blood sugar levels effectively.

- Healthy Eating Patterns: Emphasize whole, nutrient-dense foods like fruits, vegetables, whole grains, lean proteins, legumes, nuts, seeds, and healthy fats while limiting added sugars, refined carbs, processed foods, trans fats, and excessive sodium to support diabetes management and heart health.

- Macronutrient Balance: Optimize macronutrient ratios (carbohydrates, proteins, fats) based on individual needs, metabolic status, blood glucose responses, insulin sensitivity, weight management goals, and cardiovascular considerations to achieve optimal nutrient balance and metabolic control.

- Fiber-Rich Choices: Include high-fiber foods (like whole grains, fruits, vegetables, legumes, seeds) in meals to promote satiety, regulate blood sugar levels, improve digestive health, lower cholesterol, and reduce cardiovascular risks associated with diabetes.

- Heart-Healthy Fats: Prioritize sources of heart-healthy fats such as monounsaturated fats (from olive oil, avocados, nuts) and omega-3 fatty acids (from fatty fish, flaxseeds, chia seeds) while minimizing saturated fats, trans fats, and hydrogenated fats that can exacerbate inflammation, insulin resistance, and heart disease risks in individuals with diabetes.

- Glycemic Control Strategies:

- Carbohydrate Management: Implement carbohydrate counting, glycemic index/load awareness, portion control, meal timing, and consistent carbohydrate intake to regulate blood sugar levels, reduce postprandial spikes, and optimize insulin management.

- Balanced Meals and Snacks: Plan balanced meals/snacks that combine carbohydrates with proteins, healthy fats, fiber-rich foods, and low-glycemic options to achieve sustained energy, stable blood glucose, and satiety throughout the day.

- Blood Glucose Monitoring: Monitor blood glucose levels regularly, follow recommended testing protocols, track trends, adjust insulin/oral medications as needed, and collaborate with healthcare providers to achieve target ranges and prevent hyperglycemia/hypoglycemia episodes.

- **Heart-Healthy Eating Patterns:**

- Mediterranean-Inspired Diet: Adopt Mediterranean diet principles, including abundant fruits, vegetables, whole grains, legumes, nuts, seeds, olive oil, fatty fish, lean proteins, herbs, spices, and moderate wine consumption, for heart-healthy benefits, inflammation reduction, and lipid balance.

- DASH Diet Modifications: Customize DASH diet recommendations to align with diabetes management goals, emphasizing whole foods, low-sodium options, lean proteins, fiber-rich choices, healthy fats, and balanced meals/snacks to support blood pressure control and cardiovascular health.

- Low-Glycemic Choices: Choose low-glycemic index/load foods (like non-starchy vegetables, whole grains, legumes, nuts, seeds, and selected fruits) to minimize blood sugar fluctuations, improve glycemic control, reduce insulin demand, and enhance metabolic stability.

- Portion Control and Mindful Eating: Practice portion control, mindful eating, hunger/fullness awareness, mindful meal planning, and mindful snacking to avoid overeating, manage calorie intake, regulate blood sugar responses, and promote satiety cues.

- **Nutrient-Dense Foods:**

- Lean Proteins: Include lean protein sources such as poultry, fish, seafood, tofu, tempeh, legumes, and low-fat dairy products in meals to support muscle health, satiety, metabolic function, and blood sugar regulation without excessive saturated fats or cholesterol.

- Complex Carbohydrates: Choose complex carbohydrates like whole grains, fruits, vegetables, and legumes over refined carbs and sugary foods to provide sustained energy, dietary fiber, vitamins, minerals, antioxidants, and gradual blood sugar release.

- Heart-Healthy Fats: Opt for sources of heart-healthy fats such as avocados, olives, olive oil, nuts, seeds, and fatty fish (like salmon, trout) to supply essential fatty acids, monounsaturated fats, polyunsaturated fats, and antioxidants that benefit heart health, inflammation reduction, and lipid profiles.

- Antioxidant-Rich Foods: Incorporate antioxidant-rich foods like berries, citrus fruits, leafy greens, cruciferous vegetables, tomatoes, bell peppers, nuts, seeds, and dark chocolate to combat oxidative stress, support immune function, protect against cellular damage, and enhance overall health.

- **Meal Planning and Prep:**

- Personalized Nutrition Plans: Tailor nutrition plans to individual preferences, dietary restrictions, cultural considerations, and health goals, collaborating with registered dietitians, certified diabetes educators, and healthcare providers for personalized guidance and support.

- Balanced Meal Combinations: Create balanced meal combinations that include carbohydrates, proteins, healthy fats, fiber, vitamins, minerals, and fluids to meet nutritional needs, optimize blood glucose control, and promote overall well-being.

- Batch Cooking and Healthy Swaps: Practice batch cooking, meal prepping, and healthy swaps (like whole grains instead of refined grains, lean proteins instead of processed meats, plant-based fats instead of saturated fats) to streamline meal preparation, encourage healthier choices, and enhance nutrient intake.

- Mindful Eating Practices: Foster mindful eating practices, mindful meal times, mindful portioning, mindful snacking, and mindful food choices to cultivate awareness, appreciation, enjoyment, and satisfaction with meals, fostering a positive relationship with food and eating.

Navigating Nutritional Challenges

Managing diabetes and heart health through nutrition requires ongoing education, self-management skills, behavioral changes, and lifestyle modifications. Stay informed about nutritional guidelines, monitor blood sugar levels, track dietary habits, seek professional guidance, and prioritize self-care to navigate nutritional challenges effectively and promote holistic well-being.

Supplements and Nutraceuticals for Heart Health

Enhancing Heart Health with Supplements

In addition to dietary strategies, supplements and nutraceuticals can play a complementary role in promoting heart health, managing cardiovascular risks, addressing nutrient deficiencies, and supporting overall well-being. Let's explore key supplements and their potential benefits for heart disease prevention and management.

- **Omega-3 Fatty Acids:**

- Benefits: Omega-3 fatty acids (EPA, DHA) from fish oil or algae-based supplements can reduce triglycerides, lower inflammation, improve endothelial function, support heart rhythm stability, and offer cardiovascular protection.

- Sources: Choose high-quality fish oil supplements (like wild-caught salmon, mackerel, sardine, krill oil) or algae-based supplements (suitable for vegetarians/vegans) with adequate EPA and DHA concentrations, purity, potency, and third-party testing.

- **Coenzyme Q10 (CoQ10):**

- Benefits: CoQ10 is an antioxidant that supports mitochondrial function, energy production, heart muscle strength, antioxidant defenses, and cellular health, potentially benefiting individuals with heart failure, hypertension, statin-induced deficiencies, or age-related declines in CoQ10 levels.

- Sources: Consider CoQ10 supplements (ubiquinol or ubiquinone forms) with bioavailability enhancements, divided doses for absorption, and consultation with healthcare providers for dosage recommendations and monitoring.

- **Magnesium:**

- Benefits: Magnesium plays a role in heart rhythm regulation, blood pressure management, muscle function, electrolyte balance, energy metabolism, and vascular health, potentially benefiting individuals with magnesium deficiencies, arrhythmias, hypertension, or metabolic imbalances.

- Sources: Explore magnesium supplements (like magnesium citrate, glycinate, malate) with adequate elemental magnesium content, bioavailability, tolerance, and absorption considerations based on individual needs and health status.

- **Vitamin D:**

- Benefits: Vitamin D supports bone health, immune function, calcium absorption, inflammation modulation, and cardiovascular health, potentially benefiting individuals with vitamin D deficiencies, limited sun exposure, darker skin tones, or chronic diseases.

- Sources: Consider vitamin D3 supplements (cholecalciferol) with appropriate dosages, blood level monitoring, seasonal adjustments, and healthcare provider guidance to optimize vitamin D status and support heart health.

- **Fiber Supplements:**

- Benefits: Fiber supplements (like psyllium husk, glucomannan, soluble fiber blends) can support digestive health, cholesterol management, blood sugar control, satiety, weight management, and cardiovascular benefits when dietary fiber intake is insufficient or challenging to achieve through food alone.

- Sources: Explore fiber supplements with low sugar content, natural ingredients, gradual fiber release, hydration recommendations, and integration into a balanced diet for optimal benefits.

- Antioxidants:

- Benefits: Antioxidants like vitamins C and E, beta-carotene, selenium, and polyphenols from foods or supplements can reduce oxidative stress, combat inflammation, protect against cellular damage, support heart health, and enhance cardiovascular resilience.

- Sources: Obtain antioxidants from a varied diet rich in fruits, vegetables, berries, nuts, seeds, whole grains, and antioxidant-rich beverages like green tea. Consider antioxidant supplements in consultation with healthcare providers for specific health conditions or deficiencies.

- Garlic Supplements:

- Benefits: Garlic supplements may offer cardiovascular benefits, including blood pressure reduction, cholesterol management, antiplatelet effects, antioxidant properties, and endothelial function improvements, making them a potential adjunctive therapy for heart health.

- Sources: Choose garlic supplements with standardized allicin content, odorless formulations, bioavailability enhancements, and quality assurance measures to ensure potency, efficacy, and tolerability.

- **Probiotics:**

- Benefits: Probiotics (like Lactobacillus, Bifidobacterium strains) support gut microbiome balance, digestive health, immune modulation, inflammation reduction, and metabolic health, potentially benefiting individuals with gut dysbiosis, inflammation-related conditions, or metabolic imbalances.

- Sources: Consider probiotic supplements with diverse strains, colony-forming units (CFUs), survivability, prebiotics, shelf stability, refrigeration needs, and clinical evidence supporting their efficacy for specific health outcomes.

- **Herbal Supplements:**

- Benefits: Certain herbal supplements (such as hawthorn, turmeric/curcumin, ginger, ginkgo biloba, green tea extract) may have cardioprotective effects, antioxidant properties, anti-inflammatory actions, blood pressure regulation, cholesterol-lowering benefits, or endothelial function improvements, contributing to heart health support.

- Sources: Explore herbal supplements from reputable brands, standardized formulations, quality control practices, safety profiles, evidence-based dosages, and potential interactions with medications or health conditions under healthcare provider supervision.

- **Multivitamin-Mineral Supplements:**

- Benefits: Multivitamin-mineral supplements can fill nutritional gaps, support overall health, provide essential vitamins, minerals, and micronutrients, and complement dietary intake, especially for individuals with restricted diets, nutrient deficiencies, or increased nutrient needs due to age, health conditions, or lifestyle factors.

- Sources: Choose multivitamin-mineral supplements with appropriate nutrient combinations, bioavailability considerations, nutrient forms (like methylated B vitamins), elemental content, synergistic nutrients, and adherence to recommended daily allowances (RDAs) or dietary reference intakes (DRIs).

Supplement Considerations and Precautions

While supplements can offer potential benefits for heart health, it's essential to approach supplementation with caution, awareness, and informed decision-making:

- **Individualized Needs:** Consult healthcare providers, registered dietitians, or integrative medicine specialists to assess individual nutritional needs, health goals, medical history, medication interactions, nutrient status, and personalized supplement recommendations.

- **Quality and Purity:** Select supplements from reputable brands, third-party tested products, Good Manufacturing Practices (GMP) certified facilities, and quality assurance measures to ensure potency, purity, safety, and efficacy.

- **Dosage and Timing:** Follow recommended dosage guidelines, dosing schedules, timing instructions (with meals or on an empty stomach), and healthcare provider recommendations to optimize supplement absorption, minimize side effects, and achieve desired health outcomes.

- **Monitoring and Evaluation:** Monitor supplement usage, assess health improvements, track biomarkers, and conduct periodic evaluations with healthcare providers to adjust dosages, address concerns, monitor interactions, and ensure ongoing safety and efficacy.

- **Potential Interactions:** Be aware of potential supplement-drug interactions, nutrient imbalances, contraindications, allergic reactions, and adverse effects, especially when combining supplements with medications, herbs, or other dietary interventions.

- **Holistic Approach:** Supplement use should complement, not replace, a balanced diet, healthy lifestyle practices, physical activity, stress management, sleep hygiene, and regular medical care as part of a holistic approach to heart health and overall well-being.

Mind-Body Practices for Heart Health

Harmonizing Heart and Mind

Mind-body practices encompass a spectrum of techniques, therapies, and lifestyle approaches that integrate mental, emotional, physical, and spiritual dimensions to promote holistic well-being, stress resilience, relaxation, self-awareness, and heart-healthy habits. Let's explore key mind-body practices and their potential benefits for heart health.

- **Meditation and Mindfulness:**

- Benefits: Meditation and mindfulness practices cultivate present-moment awareness, focused attention, emotional regulation, stress reduction, relaxation response activation, heart rate variability improvements, and psychological well-being, contributing to heart health support.

- Techniques: Explore mindfulness meditation, guided imagery, body scan, breath awareness, loving-kindness meditation, transcendental meditation, Zen meditation, or mindfulness-based stress reduction (MBSR) programs to develop mindfulness skills, enhance resilience, and foster a positive mindset for managing stress, anxiety, depression, and emotional factors impacting heart health.

- **Yoga and Tai Chi:**

- **Benefits:** Yoga and Tai Chi blend movement, breathwork, mindfulness, flexibility, strength, balance, relaxation, and mind-body connection, offering cardiovascular benefits, stress reduction, blood pressure control, inflammation reduction, and improved mental well-being.

- **Practices:** Engage in Hatha yoga, Vinyasa flow, Iyengar yoga, Kundalini yoga, restorative yoga, Yin yoga, or therapeutic yoga sequences tailored to heart health, incorporating asanas, pranayama, meditation, and relaxation techniques.

- **Tai Chi:** Explore Tai Chi forms, Qigong exercises, Tai Chi Chuan, Taijiquan practices, or mind-body martial arts sessions focusing on slow, deliberate movements, postural alignment, mindfulness, energy flow, and relaxation for heart-centered benefits.

- **Breathwork and Relaxation Techniques:**

- **Benefits:** Breathwork techniques (like diaphragmatic breathing, box breathing, paced breathing, alternate nostril breathing) and relaxation practices (such as progressive muscle relaxation, autogenic training, visualization, biofeedback) promote stress relief, anxiety reduction, parasympathetic nervous system activation, heart rate variability improvement, and emotional balance.

- **Applications:** Incorporate breathwork and relaxation into daily routines, mindfulness practices, pre-sleep rituals, stress management strategies, workplace breaks, or guided sessions led by experienced instructors, therapists, or wellness coaches.

- **Cognitive-Behavioral Therapy (CBT):**

- **Benefits:** Cognitive-behavioral therapy (CBT) techniques address thought patterns, beliefs, emotions, behaviors, coping strategies, stress triggers, and psychological factors impacting heart health, offering tools for stress management, resilience building, emotion regulation, and positive mindset cultivation.

- **Interventions**: Explore CBT interventions, stress reduction programs, resilience training, mindfulness-based cognitive therapy (MBCT), stress inoculation training, cognitive restructuring, relaxation training, or psychoeducation sessions with qualified therapists, counselors, or psychologists.

- **Emotional Well-Being Practices:**

- **Benefits**: Emotional well-being practices encompass self-care, self-compassion, gratitude, positive psychology, social connections, emotional expression, creative outlets, meaningful activities, and lifestyle factors that nurture mental health, social support, resilience, and overall well-being.

- **Strategies**: Cultivate emotional well-being through journaling, gratitude practices, expressive arts (like music, art, dance), nature immersion, volunteer work, community engagement, hobbies, leisure activities, meaningful relationships, supportive networks, and mental health resources.

Integrating Mind-Body Practices

Integrating mind-body practices into daily life involves commitment, consistency, experimentation, and personalized exploration to find techniques that resonate and support heart health:

- **Start Slow:** Begin with small, manageable steps, gradual progress, and realistic expectations when incorporating mind-body practices into routines to build confidence, motivation, and sustainable habits over time.

- **Explore Variety:** Explore diverse mind-body techniques, classes, workshops, apps, online resources, books, videos, or community programs to discover what resonates with your preferences, needs, interests, and comfort level.

- **Seek Guidance:** Consult experienced instructors, certified practitioners, licensed therapists, or healthcare providers for guidance, personalized recommendations, skill-building strategies, and safe implementation of mind-body practices tailored to your health goals and circumstances.

- **Practice Consistency:** Establish a consistent practice schedule, daily rituals, reminders, accountability structures, or supportive environments that promote regular engagement, habit formation, and ongoing benefits from mind-body interventions.

- **Listen to Your Body:** Honor your body's cues, limitations, energy levels, and feedback during mind-body practices, adjusting intensity, duration, techniques, or modifications as needed to ensure safety, comfort, and enjoyment.

- **Reflect and Adapt:** Reflect on your experiences, progress, challenges, insights, and outcomes from mind-body practices, adapting approaches, exploring new avenues, seeking feedback, and celebrating milestones in your journey toward heart-centered well-being.

Physical Activity and Exercise for Heart Health

Energizing Heart Fitness

Physical activity and exercise are cornerstone pillars of heart health, promoting cardiovascular fitness, endurance, strength, flexibility, circulation, weight management, mood enhancement, stress resilience, and overall well-being. Let's explore the importance of physical activity for heart health and key exercise guidelines for optimal cardiovascular benefits.

- **Benefits of Physical Activity:**

- **Cardiovascular Fitness:** Regular physical activity enhances cardiovascular endurance, heart function, oxygen delivery, blood flow, cardiac output, and aerobic capacity, improving heart health, circulation, and exercise tolerance.

- **Weight Management:** Physical activity supports weight loss, weight maintenance, body composition improvements, calorie expenditure, metabolic rate enhancement, fat utilization, and energy balance for obesity prevention and heart disease risk reduction.

- **Blood Pressure Control:** Exercise contributes to lower blood pressure, improved vascular tone, endothelial function enhancement, and reduced hypertension risks through mechanisms like vasodilation, improved blood vessel elasticity, and stress reduction.

- **Blood Sugar Regulation:** Physical activity aids in glucose uptake, insulin sensitivity, glycemic control, muscle glycogen storage, postprandial glucose management, and prevention of insulin resistance, benefiting individuals with diabetes or at risk of diabetes-related heart complications.

- **Lipid Profile Improvement**: Exercise leads to favorable changes in lipid profiles, including lower LDL cholesterol levels, increased HDL cholesterol levels, reduced triglycerides, improved lipid particle size and distribution, and enhanced lipid metabolism, supporting heart health and reducing atherosclerosis risks.

- **Inflammation Reduction**: Regular exercise is associated with reduced inflammation markers (such as CRP, IL-6, TNF-alpha), oxidative stress mitigation, immune modulation, anti-inflammatory cytokine release, and cellular resilience against inflammatory stimuli, contributing to heart disease prevention and management.

- **Mental Health Benefits**: Physical activity promotes mental well-being, stress relief, mood elevation, anxiety reduction, depression management, cognitive function enhancement, sleep quality improvement, and psychosocial resilience, fostering holistic health and heart-centered lifestyle habits.

Key Exercise Guidelines for Heart Health

Effective exercise programs for heart health integrate aerobic exercise, strength training, flexibility exercises, and balance activities, tailored to individual fitness levels, health status, goals, preferences, and medical considerations:

- **Aerobic Exercise:**

  - **Type:** Engage in aerobic activities like brisk walking, jogging, running, cycling, swimming, dancing, aerobics classes, hiking, rowing, elliptical training, or sports activities that elevate heart rate, increase oxygen consumption, and improve cardiovascular fitness.

  - **Duration:** Aim for at least 150 minutes of moderate-intensity aerobic exercise per week (or 75 minutes of vigorous-intensity exercise) spread across multiple days, with gradual progression and consistency.

  - **Intensity:** Moderate-intensity exercise should feel challenging yet sustainable, with noticeable increases in breathing rate, heart rate, and perspiration, while vigorous-intensity exercise involves more significant effort and exertion, with shorter durations possible.

- **Strength Training:**

  - **Type:** Include resistance training, weightlifting, bodyweight exercises, resistance bands, or gym machines targeting major muscle groups (like legs, back, chest, shoulders, arms, core) to build strength, muscle mass, bone density, joint stability, and metabolic health.

  - **Frequency:** Perform strength training exercises at least 2-3 times per week, allowing for recovery periods between sessions and rotating muscle groups to prevent overuse injuries.

  - **Intensity:** Use appropriate weights or resistance levels that allow for 8-12 repetitions per set with proper form and technique, gradually increasing resistance, sets, or repetitions as strength improves.

- **Flexibility Exercises:**

  - **Type:** Incorporate stretching, yoga, Pilates, tai chi, mobility drills, or dynamic stretching routines to improve flexibility, joint range of motion, muscle elasticity, posture, relaxation, and injury prevention.

- **Frequency:** Include flexibility exercises in your daily routine, warm-up, cool-down, or recovery sessions, holding stretches for 15-30 seconds without bouncing or forcing movements.

- **Intensity:** Stretch to a comfortable point of tension without pain, breathing deeply and evenly, relaxing into stretches, and avoiding overstretching or pushing beyond your limits.

- **Balance and Stability Activities:**

- **Type:** Practice balance exercises, proprioception drills, stability challenges, balance boards, yoga poses, single-leg stands, or functional movements that enhance coordination, equilibrium, spatial awareness, and fall prevention.

- **Frequency:** Integrate balance and stability activities into workouts, daily activities, recreational pursuits, or specialized programs for older adults or individuals with balance impairments.

  - **Intensity**: Focus on controlled movements, steady postures, core engagement, visual fixation points, gradual progression, and safety precautions to improve balance skills safely.

Exercise Safety and Considerations

When engaging in physical activity for heart health, prioritize safety, gradual progression, proper form, hydration, warm-up, cool-down, and monitoring of signs or symptoms:

- **Health Assessment**: Consult healthcare providers, cardiologists, or exercise physiologists for pre-exercise evaluations, risk assessments, exercise prescriptions, stress testing, ECG monitoring, or personalized recommendations based on medical history, cardiovascular risks, medications, and fitness goals.

- **Cardiac Rehabilitation**: Consider cardiac rehabilitation programs for structured, supervised exercise, education, lifestyle counseling, risk factor management, peer support, and post-cardiac event recovery under medical supervision.

- **Exercise Prescription**: Follow individualized exercise prescriptions, target heart rate zones, perceived exertion scales, intensity guidelines (like METs, RPE), progression plans, and modifications as recommended by healthcare providers or exercise professionals.

- **Monitoring Symptoms:** Be aware of warning signs or symptoms during exercise, such as chest pain, palpitations, dizziness, shortness of breath, excessive fatigue, nausea, sweating, or unusual discomfort, and seek medical attention if experiencing any concerning symptoms.

- **Hydration and Nutrition:** Stay hydrated before, during, and after exercise, consume balanced meals/snacks, electrolyte-rich fluids, nutrient-dense foods, and adequate fuel to support energy levels, hydration status, muscle recovery, and exercise performance.

- **Rest and Recovery:** Allow for adequate rest, recovery, sleep, stress management, and relaxation practices between workouts to prevent overtraining, fatigue, burnout, injuries, and optimize adaptation, fitness gains, and overall well-being.

Incorporating Movement into Daily Life

Beyond structured exercise sessions, prioritize daily movement, active lifestyle habits, and physical activity integration into daily routines:

- **Active Commuting**: Walk, bike, use public transportation, or incorporate active commuting options into your daily travel to increase steps, movement, and physical activity throughout the day.

- **Workplace Movement**: Take breaks, stand up, stretch, walk around, use standing desks, perform desk exercises, engage in brief movement breaks, or organize walking meetings to combat sedentary behavior and promote circulation.

- **Household Chores**: Turn household chores into physical activity opportunities by gardening, cleaning, vacuuming, mopping, organizing, lifting, carrying, or performing tasks that involve movement, muscle engagement, and calorie expenditure.

- **Recreational Activities**: Engage in recreational sports, outdoor activities, leisure pursuits, hobbies, dancing, social gatherings, or group classes that combine enjoyment, social interaction, and physical movement for holistic health benefits.

Long-Term Lifestyle Commitment

Maintaining heart-healthy habits requires long-term commitment and consistency. Here are some key strategies for integrating heart-healthy practices into your long-term lifestyle:

1. Goal Setting and Planning: Set specific, measurable, achievable, relevant, and time-bound (SMART) goals related to heart health, nutrition, exercise, stress management, and overall well-being. Create action plans, timelines, milestones, and strategies to track progress, adjust goals, and stay motivated.

2. Daily Heart-Healthy Choices: Make conscious choices daily that prioritize heart health, such as choosing nutrient-dense foods, practicing portion control, staying hydrated, incorporating physical activity, managing stress, getting quality sleep, and avoiding tobacco/smoking.

3. Mindful Eating Practices: Practice mindful eating by slowing down, savoring flavors, listening to hunger/fullness cues, avoiding distractions, enjoying balanced meals/snacks, practicing gratitude, and cultivating a positive relationship with food and eating.

4. Regular Physical Activity: Incorporate regular physical activity into your routine by scheduling workouts, setting reminders, trying new activities, varying exercises, seeking social support, tracking progress, celebrating achievements, and adapting workouts to fit your schedule and preferences.

5. Stress Management Techniques: Explore stress management techniques like deep breathing, meditation, mindfulness, yoga, tai chi, progressive muscle relaxation, guided imagery, journaling, hobbies, time management, and setting boundaries to reduce stress, promote relaxation, and improve resilience.

6. Social Support and Community: Build a supportive network of family, friends, peers, healthcare providers, fitness professionals, online communities, or support groups focused on heart health, wellness, motivation, accountability, encouragement, and shared experiences.

7. Regular Health Checkups: Prioritize regular health checkups, screenings, blood tests, blood pressure monitoring, cholesterol checks, diabetes screenings, medication reviews, cardiac evaluations, and follow-ups with healthcare providers for preventive care and early detection of health concerns.

8. Sleep Quality and Quantity: Prioritize sleep hygiene, consistent sleep schedules, relaxation before bedtime, comfortable sleep environment, limiting screen time, avoiding stimulants, and addressing sleep disorders to improve sleep quality, duration, and overall well-being.

9. Holistic Well-Being: Embrace a holistic approach to well-being by addressing physical, mental, emotional, social, and spiritual aspects of health through self-care practices, self-reflection, self-compassion, self-improvement, meaningful connections, purposeful living, and life balance.

10. Lifelong Learning and Adaptation: Stay informed about heart health, nutrition, exercise science, wellness trends, research advancements, evidence-based practices, and lifestyle strategies through reliable sources, continuing education, workshops, seminars, books, articles, podcasts, and professional guidance.

By integrating these strategies into your lifestyle, maintaining consistency, seeking support when needed, and staying committed to your health goals, you can cultivate long-term heart-healthy habits that contribute to a vibrant, fulfilling, and resilient life.

Chapter 4

Lifestyle and Heart Health:

1. Nutrition for Heart Health:

- **Balanced Diet**: A heart-healthy diet emphasizes whole, unprocessed foods rich in nutrients, fiber, antioxidants, and phytochemicals. Include a variety of fruits, vegetables, whole grains, lean proteins (such as poultry, fish, legumes), nuts, seeds, and healthy fats (like olive oil, avocado, fatty fish) to promote cardiovascular wellness.

- **Key Nutrients**: Prioritize nutrients essential for heart health, such as omega-3 fatty acids (from fish, flaxseeds, chia seeds), soluble fiber (found in oats, legumes, fruits), potassium (in bananas, sweet potatoes, leafy greens), magnesium (from nuts, seeds, whole grains), and antioxidants (from colorful fruits/vegetables, berries, nuts).

- **Heart-Healthy Eating Patterns:** Consider adopting eating patterns like the Mediterranean diet, DASH (Dietary Approaches to Stop Hypertension) diet, plant-based diet, or mindful eating approach that emphasize plant foods, limit processed foods, reduce sodium/sugar intake, and promote mindful, enjoyable eating experiences.

- **Sodium Reduction:** Monitor sodium intake by reading food labels, choosing low-sodium options, minimizing added salt in cooking/preparation, using herbs/spices for flavor, avoiding processed foods, and limiting high-sodium condiments, sauces, and snacks to manage blood pressure and heart health.

- **Sugar and Saturated Fat Control:** Limit added sugars, sugary beverages, desserts, refined carbohydrates, trans fats, saturated fats (found in red meat, full-fat dairy, fried foods) to lower cholesterol levels, improve lipid profiles, reduce inflammation, and support heart disease prevention.

- **Meal Planning and Portion Control:** Plan balanced meals/snacks, practice portion control, eat mindfully, listen to hunger/fullness cues, avoid oversized portions, use smaller plates/bowls, and focus on nutrient density, quality, variety, and mindful eating habits for long-term heart wellness.

2. Physical Activity for Heart Health:

- **Aerobic Exercise:** Engage in aerobic activities (like walking, jogging, cycling, swimming, dancing) that elevate heart rate, improve cardiovascular fitness, increase oxygen delivery, enhance circulation, and boost energy levels for overall heart health.

- **Strength Training:** Incorporate resistance training, weightlifting, bodyweight exercises, or gym workouts targeting major muscle groups to build strength, endurance, muscle mass, bone density, metabolism, and functional fitness for heart disease prevention.

- **Flexibility and Balance:** Include flexibility exercises (like stretching, yoga) and balance activities (such as tai chi, stability exercises) to improve joint mobility, range of motion, posture, stability, coordination, fall prevention, and overall physical function.

- **Exercise Guidelines**: Follow recommended exercise guidelines, such as 150 minutes of moderate-intensity aerobic exercise per week, strength training sessions 2-3 times weekly, flexibility/balance activities regularly, warm-up/cool-down routines, and gradual progression in intensity/duration.

- **Cardiovascular Workouts**: Incorporate cardiovascular workouts like interval training, circuit training, HIIT (high-intensity interval training), cardio classes, outdoor activities, sports, or group fitness sessions for variety, motivation, challenge, and heart-healthy benefits.

- **Consistency and Variety**: Maintain consistency in your exercise routine, mix up workouts to prevent boredom, plateaus, or overuse injuries, listen to your body, adjust intensity as needed, stay hydrated, wear appropriate gear, and seek guidance from fitness professionals for safe, effective workouts.

3. Stress Management for Heart Health:

- **Stress Awareness:** Recognize sources of stress (such as work, relationships, finances, health concerns) and their impact on physical, mental, and emotional well-being, noting signs/symptoms of stress like muscle tension, headaches, insomnia, anxiety, irritability.

- **Stress Reduction Techniques:** Practice stress reduction techniques like deep breathing, relaxation exercises, meditation, mindfulness, progressive muscle relaxation, guided imagery, visualization, or biofeedback to activate the relaxation response, calm the mind, and reduce physiological stress responses.

- **Mindfulness Practices:** Cultivate mindfulness through present-moment awareness, non-judgmental observation, acceptance of thoughts/feelings, gratitude practices, mindful eating, sensory awareness, mindful movement (like yoga, tai chi), and daily mindfulness routines to enhance resilience and emotional balance.

- **Healthy Coping Strategies:** Develop healthy coping strategies for stress management, such as time management, prioritizing tasks, setting realistic goals, delegating responsibilities, problem-solving, seeking social support, expressing emotions, practicing self-care, and maintaining a positive outlook.

- **Stress Reduction Activities:** Engage in stress-relieving activities like hobbies, creative outlets, nature walks, journaling, music therapy, aromatherapy, laughter/yoga therapy, relaxation techniques, self-compassion practices, or relaxation-inducing rituals to promote relaxation, self-care, and stress resilience.

- **Lifestyle Modifications:** Make lifestyle modifications to reduce chronic stress, such as setting boundaries, limiting exposure to stressors, improving work-life balance, practicing assertiveness, seeking professional support/counseling, and adopting stress-reducing habits for long-term heart health.

4. Quality Sleep and Heart Health:

- **Sleep Hygiene:** Practice good sleep hygiene habits, such as maintaining a consistent sleep schedule, creating a relaxing bedtime routine, minimizing screen time (phones, computers, TVs), keeping the bedroom dark/quiet/comfortable, and avoiding stimulants (caffeine, nicotine) close to bedtime.

- **Sleep Duration:** Aim for 7-9 hours of quality sleep per night for adults to support physical recovery, cognitive function, emotional regulation, hormone balance, immune function, memory consolidation, and cardiovascular health.

- **Sleep Disorders:** Address sleep disorders (like insomnia, sleep apnea, restless legs syndrome) promptly through medical evaluation, diagnosis, treatment, lifestyle modifications, sleep studies, CPAP therapy, dental appliances, weight management, positional therapy, or behavioral interventions.

- **Sleep Tracking and Improvement:** Use sleep tracking tools, apps, wearables, or journals to monitor sleep patterns, identify sleep disturbances, track sleep quality/quantity, assess sleep hygiene practices, and make adjustments for better sleep habits and overall heart wellness.

- **Sleep-Heart Connection:** Understand the link between sleep and heart health, as quality sleep supports heart rhythm regulation, blood pressure control, inflammation reduction, stress hormone balance, metabolic function, cardiovascular recovery, and overall cardiovascular resilience.

5. Tobacco Cessation and Heart Health:

- **Smoking Risks:** Acknowledge the risks of smoking and tobacco use on heart health, including increased heart disease risk, atherosclerosis, hypertension, stroke, heart attacks, peripheral artery disease, coronary artery disease, arrhythmias, and cardiovascular complications.

- **Benefits of Quitting:** Recognize the immediate and long-term benefits of quitting smoking, such as improved circulation, reduced heart disease risk, lower blood pressure, decreased inflammation, enhanced lung function, better oxygen delivery, and decreased risk of smoking-related illnesses.

6. Alcohol Moderation and Heart Health:

- **Moderate Consumption:** If consuming alcohol, do so in moderation and adhere to recommended limits (such as up to one drink per day for women and up to two drinks per day for men) to minimize cardiovascular risks, liver damage, hypertension, cardiomyopathy, arrhythmias, and alcohol-related health issues.

- **Alcohol Guidelines**: Follow guidelines for responsible alcohol consumption, avoid binge drinking, excessive drinking, heavy drinking, or high-risk drinking patterns, monitor alcohol intake, stay hydrated, eat before drinking, and consider alcohol-free days to maintain heart health and overall well-being.

- **Health Impact**: Be aware of the health impact of alcohol on heart health, blood pressure, cholesterol levels, triglycerides, heart rhythm disturbances, heart muscle function, clotting factors, stroke risk, heart failure, and interactions with medications or existing health conditions.

7. Social Connection and Heart Health:

- **Social Support Network**: Cultivate strong social connections, supportive relationships, friendships, family bonds, and community ties that promote emotional well-being, stress resilience, happiness, laughter, companionship, empathy, communication, and shared experiences.

- **Isolation Risks:** Recognize the risks of social isolation, loneliness, lack of social support, or disconnectedness on mental health, emotional balance, stress coping, immune function, inflammation, cardiovascular health, and overall mortality risks.

- **Social Engagement:** Participate in social activities, group settings, social clubs, volunteer work, community events, team sports, hobby groups, religious gatherings, or online communities to foster social interaction, belongingness, networking, and emotional support for heart health.

- **Communication Skills:** Enhance communication skills, active listening, empathy, assertiveness, conflict resolution, social skills, emotional intelligence, and relationship-building abilities to nurture healthy connections, resolve conflicts, express feelings, and maintain positive social interactions.

8. Financial Health and Stress Reduction:

- **Financial Management**: Practice responsible financial management, budgeting, saving, debt management, financial planning, investment strategies, emergency funds, retirement planning, insurance coverage, and financial literacy to reduce financial stress, anxiety, and uncertainty.

- **Financial Stress Impact**: Acknowledge the impact of financial stress on mental health, emotional well-being, relationships, sleep quality, productivity, decision-making, physical health, coping strategies, and overall stress management.

- **Stress Reduction Techniques**: Use stress reduction techniques like financial planning, goal setting, prioritizing expenses, seeking financial advice, creating financial buffers, avoiding impulsive spending, negotiating debts, and developing healthy money habits to improve financial wellness and reduce stress.

9. Emotional Health and Well-Being:

- **Emotional Awareness**:

Develop emotional awareness, self-awareness, emotional regulation, mindfulness, self-reflection, and self-compassion practices to understand and manage emotions, thoughts, behaviors, stress responses, triggers, and coping mechanisms.

- **Positive Emotions:** Cultivate positive emotions like gratitude, optimism, joy, humor, resilience, kindness, forgiveness, acceptance, and humor to promote emotional well-being, psychological resilience, stress resilience, and overall life satisfaction.

- **Mental Health Support:** Seek mental health support, therapy, counseling, psychotherapy, support groups, or professional help when needed to address mental health concerns, emotional challenges, mood disorders, anxiety, depression, trauma, grief, or life transitions impacting heart health and well-being.

10. Environmental Health Considerations:

- **Environmental Awareness:**

Be mindful of environmental factors that impact heart health, such as air quality, pollution, allergens, toxins, chemicals, workplace hazards, indoor air quality, water quality, climate conditions, and environmental exposures that may affect cardiovascular function.

   - *Environmental Modifications:* Make environmental modifications, improvements, or adjustments to create a healthier living/work environment, reduce exposure to pollutants, allergens, irritants, carcinogens, and toxins, and promote respiratory health, cardiovascular health, and overall well-being.

By incorporating these lifestyle practices, healthy habits, and holistic approaches into your daily life, you can support heart health, reduce cardiovascular risks, promote overall wellness, and enhance your quality of life.

Chapter 5

Emerging Advancements in Heart Cardiology

1. Precision Medicine in Cardiology:

- **Genomic Testing**: Explore the role of genomic testing, genetic screening, DNA analysis, and personalized medicine in identifying genetic predispositions, inherited heart conditions, familial risk factors, pharmacogenomics, and targeted treatment approaches.

- **Biomarker Assessment**: Utilize biomarker assessments, molecular diagnostics, blood tests, inflammatory markers, lipid profiles, cardiac enzymes, troponin levels, B-type natriuretic peptide (BNP), C-reactive protein (CRP), and other biomarkers for risk stratification, early detection, prognosis prediction, and treatment monitoring.

- **Precision Therapies**: Implement precision therapies, individualized treatment plans, genotype-specific medications, gene-based interventions, molecular targets, gene editing techniques, stem cell therapies, and gene therapies for cardiovascular diseases, arrhythmias, heart failure, inherited cardiomyopathies, and congenital heart defects.

2. Artificial Intelligence (AI) and Machine Learning (ML) in Cardiology:

- **AI Algorithms:** Harness AI algorithms, machine learning models, predictive analytics, deep learning, natural language processing, data mining, and pattern recognition to analyze vast datasets, electronic health records (EHRs), imaging studies, genetic data, wearable device data, and clinical variables for early disease detection, risk assessment, treatment optimization, and decision support.

- **Clinical Decision Support:** Integrate AI-driven clinical decision support systems, predictive risk scores, risk calculators, diagnostic tools, treatment algorithms, virtual health assistants, telemedicine platforms, and remote monitoring solutions into cardiology practice for personalized patient care, real-time insights, and evidence-based interventions.

- **Image Analysis:** Use AI-based image analysis, computer-aided detection/diagnosis, image recognition, radiomics, echocardiography algorithms, cardiac MRI/CT image interpretation, and automated image processing for accurate diagnostics, lesion detection, cardiac function assessment, and imaging-guided interventions.

3. Telecardiology and Remote Monitoring:

- **Teleconsultations:** Embrace teleconsultations, virtual visits, telemedicine platforms, video conferencing, remote patient monitoring, and digital health technologies for cardiology consultations, follow-ups, second opinions, medication management, lifestyle counseling, and patient education.

- **Home Monitoring Devices:** Utilize home monitoring devices, wearable sensors, smartwatches, mobile apps, ECG monitors, blood pressure cuffs, implantable devices (like pacemakers, defibrillators), and continuous monitoring systems for real-time data collection, cardiac rhythm analysis, symptom tracking, medication adherence, and early intervention.

- **Data Integration:** Integrate telecardiology data, remote monitoring data, patient-reported outcomes, device-generated data, wearables data, electronic health records, lab results, imaging studies, and healthcare analytics into centralized platforms, electronic platforms, or health information systems for comprehensive care coordination, clinical insights, and collaborative decision-making.

4. Regenerative Medicine and Stem Cell Therapies:

- **Cell-Based Therapies:** Explore regenerative medicine approaches, stem cell therapies, cell-based treatments, tissue engineering, cardiac regeneration strategies, myocardial repair techniques, and vascular regeneration interventions for heart tissue repair, functional recovery, scar reduction, and cardiac remodeling.

- **Stem Cell Sources:** Investigate various stem cell sources, including bone marrow-derived stem cells, adipose-derived stem cells, cardiac progenitor cells, induced pluripotent stem cells (iPSCs), mesenchymal stem cells (MSCs), and stem cell transplantation techniques for myocardial infarction, heart failure, cardiomyopathy, and ischemic heart disease.

   - **Clinical Trials:** Stay updated on ongoing clinical trials, research studies, preclinical models, translational research, regenerative medicine protocols, stem cell safety/efficacy assessments, patient outcomes, long-term follow-ups, regulatory approvals, and ethical considerations in stem cell therapies for cardiovascular disorders.

5. Gene Editing and CRISPR Technology in Cardiology:

   - **CRISPR-Cas9 System:** Understand the CRISPR-Cas9 gene editing system, gene modification techniques, genome engineering tools, gene correction strategies, and CRISPR applications in targeting genetic mutations, modifying DNA sequences, editing gene expression, and correcting hereditary cardiac conditions.

   - **Genome Modifications:** Explore potential genome modifications, gene therapies, gene silencing approaches, gene knockout techniques, gene insertion/deletion methods, and CRISPR-based interventions for treating genetic heart diseases, arrhythmias, hypertrophic cardiomyopathy, familial hypercholesterolemia, and other inherited cardiovascular disorders.

- **Ethical and Safety Considerations**: Address ethical dilemmas, safety concerns, off-target effects, immune responses, long-term risks, regulatory frameworks, patient consent, informed decision-making, and societal implications associated with gene editing technologies, genome engineering, and genetic interventions in cardiology practice.

6. Nanotechnology and Drug Delivery Systems:

- **Nanoparticle Therapeutics**: Explore nanotechnology applications, nanoparticle drug delivery systems, nanomedicine platforms, nano-sized drug carriers, targeted drug delivery strategies, and nanoscale interventions for cardiovascular drug delivery, localized therapies, site-specific action, reduced side effects, and enhanced treatment efficacy.

- **Smart Nanomaterials**: Investigate smart nanomaterials, nanosensors, nanodevices, nanocarriers, nanobiomaterials, and nanotechnology-enabled approaches for drug release kinetics, controlled release, sustained drug delivery, tissue targeting, cellular uptake, biocompatibility, bioavailability, pharmacokinetics, pharmacodynamics, and therapeutic outcomes in cardiovascular medicine.

7. Non-Invasive Imaging Technologies:

- **Advanced Imaging Modalities**: Explore non-invasive imaging technologies, advanced imaging modalities, cardiac imaging techniques, and diagnostic tools such as cardiac MRI (magnetic resonance imaging), CT (computed tomography) angiography, PET (positron emission tomography), SPECT (single-photon emission computed tomography), echocardiography, coronary calcium scoring, and cardiac CT for comprehensive cardiac assessment, structural evaluation, functional analysis, plaque detection, perfusion imaging, and early disease detection.

- **3D Imaging and Virtual Reality:** Utilize 3D imaging, virtual reality (VR), augmented reality (AR), holography, 3D reconstruction techniques, and immersive visualization platforms for anatomical modeling, surgical planning, interventional cardiology procedures, cardiac simulations, medical education, and patient engagement in cardiovascular care.

8. Cardiovascular Biotechnology and Biomaterials:

- **Biocompatible Materials:** Explore cardiovascular biotechnology, biomaterial sciences, biocompatible materials, bioengineering solutions, tissue engineering constructs, scaffolds, patches, grafts, implants, and medical devices designed for cardiac repair, regeneration, vascular interventions, and cardiac implantable technologies.

- **Tissue Engineering Approaches:** Investigate tissue engineering approaches, cellular therapies, regenerative strategies, cardiac tissue constructs, engineered blood vessels, organ-on-a-chip technologies, and biofabrication methods for creating functional cardiac tissues, vascular grafts, cardiac patches, and bioartificial organs in cardiac medicine.

9. Digital Health Innovations:

- **Health Information Technology**: Embrace digital health innovations, health information technology (HIT), electronic medical records (EMRs), health data analytics, remote monitoring platforms, patient portals, mobile health apps, wearable sensors, health informatics, and telehealth solutions for efficient data management, real-time monitoring, patient engagement, health outcomes tracking, and telecardiology services.

- **Healthcare AI and Analytics**: Leverage healthcare AI, predictive analytics, big data analytics, machine learning algorithms, clinical decision support tools, population health management systems, and data-driven insights for evidence-based medicine, risk prediction, treatment optimization, disease management, patient stratification, and healthcare quality improvement in cardiology.

10. Regulatory Advances and Clinical Trials:

- **Regulatory Frameworks:** Stay informed about regulatory advances, guidelines, regulatory pathways, quality standards, ethical considerations, regulatory approvals, clinical trial regulations, and compliance requirements governing cardiovascular therapies, medical devices, digital health technologies, and innovative treatments.

- **Clinical Trial Landscape:** Monitor the clinical trial landscape, research studies, randomized controlled trials (RCTs), multi-center trials, observational studies, real-world evidence, post-market surveillance, long-term safety/efficacy assessments, patient outcomes, health economics, and comparative effectiveness research in cardiovascular medicine.

11. Patient-Centered Care and Shared Decision-Making:

- **Patient Engagement:** Promote patient-centered care, shared decision-making, patient empowerment, health literacy, patient education, informed consent, personalized medicine, patient preferences, treatment choices, and collaborative care models that involve patients in their healthcare decisions, treatment plans, and self-management strategies.

- **Patient Advocacy:** Advocate for patient rights, patient safety, patient advocacy, patient support programs, patient education initiatives, patient advocacy organizations, patient-centered initiatives, patient feedback mechanisms, and patient-provider partnerships that prioritize patient well-being, satisfaction, dignity, and holistic care in cardiology practice.

12. Global Health Initiatives and Collaborations:

- **International Collaborations:** Foster global health initiatives, international collaborations, cross-border research, knowledge exchange, scientific partnerships, global health equity, capacity-building programs, public health interventions, and collaborative efforts to address cardiovascular disease burden, disparities, and global health challenges.

- **Public Health Policies**: Advocate for public health policies, cardiovascular prevention programs, health promotion campaigns, lifestyle interventions, community outreach, education campaigns, screening initiatives, early detection strategies, and policy interventions aimed at reducing cardiovascular risk factors, promoting heart-healthy behaviors, and improving population health outcomes worldwide.

By exploring these emerging advancements, technological innovations, research breakthroughs, regulatory landscapes, patient-centered approaches, and global collaborations in cardiovascular medicine, we can continue to advance heart health, enhance clinical care, improve patient outcomes, and transform the landscape of cardiovascular medicine.

13. Ethical Considerations in Cardiovascular Research and Practice:

- **Ethical Framework**: Discuss ethical considerations, principles of medical ethics, patient rights, privacy issues, confidentiality, informed consent, beneficence, non-maleficence, justice, autonomy, and professional integrity in cardiovascular research, clinical trials, patient care, and healthcare decision-making.

- **Research Ethics:** Address ethical challenges, conflicts of interest, research misconduct, data integrity, research transparency, publication ethics, authorship guidelines, peer review processes, conflicts resolution mechanisms, and ethical standards governing cardiovascular research.

- **Patient-Centered Ethics:** Emphasize patient-centered ethics, cultural competence, diversity considerations, healthcare disparities, vulnerable populations, patient advocacy, shared decision-making, patient autonomy, respect for patient preferences, and ethical dilemmas in clinical practice.

14. Cardiovascular Education and Training:

- **Medical Education:** Highlight cardiovascular education, training programs, medical curriculum enhancements, continuing medical education (CME), professional development, competency-based training, simulation training, hands-on workshops, case-based learning, and interdisciplinary training in cardiology, cardiac surgery, electrophysiology, interventional cardiology, imaging, and cardiovascular nursing.

   - **Digital Learning:** Integrate digital learning platforms, online resources, virtual simulations, e-learning modules, webinars, virtual conferences, tele-education, tele-mentoring, and mobile learning tools for remote education, skill development, knowledge sharing, and lifelong learning in cardiovascular healthcare.

15. Patient Safety and Quality Improvement:

   - **Patient Safety Initiatives:** Implement patient safety initiatives, quality improvement projects, patient safety protocols, error reporting systems, adverse event monitoring, medication safety measures, infection control practices, surgical safety checklists, and evidence-based guidelines to enhance patient safety, reduce medical errors, prevent complications, and improve healthcare outcomes in cardiology.

- **Quality Metrics**: Monitor quality metrics, performance indicators, outcome measures, benchmarking data, quality assessment tools, risk-adjusted outcomes, patient satisfaction surveys, healthcare accreditation standards, and quality improvement initiatives to evaluate healthcare quality, track progress, identify areas for improvement, and promote continuous quality enhancement in cardiovascular care.

16. Healthcare Innovations and Disruptive Technologies:

- **Digital Disruption**: Explore healthcare innovations, disruptive technologies, digital transformation, health tech startups, telehealth platforms, wearable devices, remote monitoring solutions, artificial intelligence, machine learning, blockchain applications, big data analytics, and precision medicine tools driving innovation in cardiovascular healthcare delivery, patient outcomes, data management, and healthcare efficiency.

- **Healthcare Entrepreneurship:** Encourage healthcare entrepreneurship, innovation ecosystems, startup incubators, venture capital funding, industry collaborations, technology transfer, intellectual property protection, regulatory compliance, market adoption, and commercialization pathways for cardiovascular innovations, medical devices, digital health solutions, and novel therapies.

17. Global Cardiac Health Initiatives:

- **Global Health Partnerships:** Foster global cardiac health initiatives, public-private partnerships, international collaborations, nonprofit organizations, philanthropic initiatives, humanitarian missions, medical volunteering, capacity-building programs, health education campaigns, and advocacy efforts to address global cardiovascular disease burden, promote heart health awareness, and improve cardiac care access, affordability, and equity worldwide.

- *Healthcare Sustainability:* Address healthcare sustainability, resource allocation, healthcare disparities, social determinants of health, access to care issues, universal health coverage, health equity, financial barriers, affordability challenges, and policy advocacy for sustainable healthcare systems, equitable healthcare delivery, and cardiovascular health equity on a global scale.

By delving into these diverse areas of cardiovascular medicine, exploring cutting-edge advancements, embracing ethical principles, promoting education and training, prioritizing patient safety and quality improvement, fostering innovation and collaboration, and advocating for global cardiac health initiatives, we can continue to advance the field, improve patient outcomes, and create a healthier future for individuals with cardiovascular conditions.

Chapter 6

Medical Interventions And Innovations

Heart disease remains a global health concern, claiming millions of lives each year. However, the fight against this formidable foe is far from over. The medical field is constantly innovating, developing new interventions and treatments to diagnose, prevent, and manage heart disease more effectively. Here's a glimpse into the ever-evolving arsenal against heart disease:

Traditional Medical Interventions:

- **Minimally Invasive Procedures**: Techniques like angioplasty and stenting open blocked arteries, improving blood flow to the heart.
  Angioplasty: This is a procedure to widen narrowed or blocked arteries using a balloon catheter, often followed by stent placement to keep the artery open.
  Stenting: Stenting is the placement of a small metal or plastic tube (stent) in the artery to improve blood flow and prevent re-narrowing.

- **Percutaneous Coronary Intervention (PCI):** This is a minimally invasive procedure that combines angioplasty and stenting to treat coronary artery disease (CAD) and relieve chest pain (angina).

- **Transcatheter Aortic Valve Replacement (TAVR):** TAVR is a minimally invasive alternative to open-heart surgery for replacing a narrowed aortic valve, suitable for high-risk or inoperable patients.

- **Atrial Septal Defect (ASD) Closure:** It is a minimally invasive procedure to repair a hole in the heart's septum using a device inserted through a catheter.

- *Coronary Artery Bypass Grafting (CABG):* This traditional open-heart surgery reroutes blood flow around blocked arteries using healthy vessels from other parts of the body.

- **Valve Replacement Surgery**: Damaged heart valves can be repaired or replaced with artificial valves, restoring proper blood flow.
- **Pacemakers and Defibrillators**: These implanted devices regulate the heart's rhythm, preventing potentially life-threatening arrhythmias.
- **Medications**: A variety of medications play a crucial role in managing heart disease, including cholesterol-lowering drugs, blood thinners, and blood pressure medications.

Cutting-Edge Innovations:
- **Transcatheter Aortic Valve Replacement (TAVR)**: This minimally invasive procedure replaces a narrowed aortic valve without the need for open-heart surgery.

- **Robotic-Assisted Cardiac Surgery**: Robots assist surgeons with greater precision and control during complex heart procedures.

Robotic Surgery in Cardiology:

- **- Robot-Assisted CABG**: Robot-assisted coronary artery bypass grafting (CABG) is a minimally invasive approach using robotic arms controlled by a surgeon to perform precise grafting procedures on the heart.

- **- Robotic Mitral Valve Repair**: Robotic mitral valve repair is a technique for repairing a leaky mitral valve using robotic instruments for improved precision and outcomes.

- **- Robotic Atrial Fibrillation Ablation**: Robotic atrial fibrillation ablation is a minimally invasive procedure to treat irregular heartbeats (atrial fibrillation) using robotic tools to create scar tissue in the heart's atria, restoring normal rhythm.

- **Gene Therapy**: Researchers are exploring the potential of gene therapy to modify genes associated with heart disease risk factors. Genetic testing for cardiovascular diseases, including inherited conditions such as familial hypercholesterolemia, hypertrophic cardiomyopathy, and genetic risk factors for atherosclerosis and thrombosis.

- **Precision Medicine Approaches**: Precision medicine are approaches that tailor treatment plans based on individual genetic profiles, including personalized medication regimens, risk assessments, and targeted therapies.

- **Stem Cell Therapy**: Studies are underway to investigate the use of stem cells to regenerate damaged heart tissue.

- **3D Printing**: This technology offers promise for creating personalized heart valves or even bioprinting tissues for repair.

Advancements in Cardiac Imaging:

- **- Cardiac MRI**: Cardiac MRI is a non-invasive imaging technique that uses magnets and radio waves to create detailed images of the heart's structure, function, and blood flow.

- **- CT Angiography**: CT angiography is a type of CT scan that produces detailed images of the heart's blood vessels, helping diagnose coronary artery disease and other vascular conditions.

- **- 3D Echocardiography**: 3D echocardiography is an advanced ultrasound technique that creates three-dimensional images of the heart, aiding in the assessment of cardiac function and abnormalities.

- **- Nuclear Imaging Techniques:** Nuclear imaging techniques such as myocardial perfusion scans and PET scans, which use radioactive tracers to evaluate blood flow, heart muscle function, and cardiac viability.

- **Telehealth And Remote Monitoring:** Remote monitoring of heart health through wearable devices and smartphone apps allows for early detection of potential problems.

- **Virtual Consultations:** Virtual consultations and telemedicine platforms allow remote access to cardiac consultations, follow-ups, and monitoring.

- **Remote Patient Monitoring:**

Remote monitoring devices, wearable sensors, and digital health technologies are used to track cardiac parameters, detect abnormalities, and improve patient outcomes.

- **Implantable Cardiac Technology**

- **Pacemakers:**

Pacemakers are implantable devices that regulate the heart's rhythm by sending electrical impulses to the heart muscle, used to treat bradycardia and other rhythm disorders.

- **Implantable Cardioverter-Defibrillators (ICDs):**

ICDs are devices that monitor heart rhythm and deliver electric shocks or pacing to treat life-threatening arrhythmias such as ventricular fibrillation.

- **Cardiac Resynchronization Therapy (CRT) Devices:** CRT devices are implantable devices that coordinate the heart's contractions to improve pumping efficiency, often used in heart failure patients with dyssynchrony.

- **Left Ventricular Assist Devices (LVADs):** LVADs are mechanical pumps implanted in the chest to assist a weakened left ventricle in pumping blood, used as a bridge to transplantation or as destination therapy in heart failure patients.

- **Artificial Heart Technology:**

- **Total Artificial Hearts (TAHs):** TAHs are mechanical devices that replace the function of the entire heart, used temporarily until a heart transplant is available.

\- **Ventricular Assist Devices (VADs):** VADs are mechanical pumps that assist the heart's pumping function, used as bridge-to-transplant or long-term therapy in heart failure patients.

- **Drug Development and Pharmacotherapy:**

\- **Novel Drug Classes:** Explore new drug classes for cardiovascular diseases, such as PCSK9 inhibitors for cholesterol management, SGLT2 inhibitors for heart failure, and novel antiplatelet agents.

\- **Targeted Therapies:** Targeted therapies are focused on specific molecular pathways in cardiovascular disorders, including anti-inflammatory drugs, endothelin receptor antagonists, and renin-angiotensin-aldosterone system (RAAS) inhibitors.

- **Emerging Therapies in Heart Failure:**

\- **Sacubitril/Valsartan (ARNI) Therapy:** ARNI therapy is a novel approach to heart management that combines neprilysin inhibition with angiotensin receptor blockade.

- **SGLT2 Inhibitors:** SGLT2 inhibitors in heart failure treatment, is beneficial in reducing heart failure hospitalizations and improving outcomes.

- **HFpEF Therapies:** Explore emerging therapies for heart failure with preserved ejection fraction (HFpEF), including diuretics, mineralocorticoid receptor antagonists, and novel investigational agents.

The Focus on Prevention:

As much as medical interventions are crucial, a significant emphasis lies on preventing heart disease altogether. Here's where lifestyle modifications come into play:

- **Healthy Diet:** Maintaining a balanced diet low in saturated fats, sodium, and added sugars is key.
- **Regular Exercise:** Aim for at least 150 minutes of moderate-intensity exercise per week.
- **Smoking Cessation:** Smoking is a major risk factor for heart disease. Quitting smoking significantly reduces the risk.

- **Weight Management**: Maintaining a healthy weight lowers the burden on the heart.
- **Stress Management**: Chronic stress can contribute to heart disease. Practice stress-relieving techniques like meditation or yoga.

The Road Ahead:

The fight against heart disease is a continuous journey. Continued research and development hold the potential for even more transformative interventions and personalized medicine approaches.

By combining traditional medical interventions with preventative measures and cutting-edge innovations, we can create a future where heart disease has a diminished impact on lives around the world.

Chapter 7

Nurturing Your Heart: A Holistic Approach to Heart Health:

Your heart is something other than a muscle that siphons blood; it's the center of your well-being, unpredictably associated with your physical, mental, and emotional state. While present day medication offers incredible resources to battle coronary illness, an all encompassing methodology that tends to all parts of your life is critical for ideal heart wellbeing. We should dive into the multi-layered universe of comprehensive heart care:

Sustaining Your Body:

- **Dietary Decisions**: Embrace a heart-sound eating routine wealthy in organic products, vegetables, entire grains, and lean proteins. Limit soaked fats, trans fats, added sugars, and handled food varieties. Investigate dietary examples like the Mediterranean eating routine, known for its heart-defensive advantages.

• **Fiber - Force to be reckoned with**: Increase your fiber intake with natural products, vegetables, beans, lentils, and entire grains. Fiber helps lower cholesterol and manage glucose, both urgent for a sound heart.

• **Solid Fats**: Not all fats are made equivalent! Incorporate sound fats from sources like avocados, nuts, seeds, and olive oil in your eating routine. These fats advance great cholesterol levels and diminish aggravation.

• **Hydration Legend**: Water is fundamental for ideal wellbeing, including heart capability. Aim to drink water day to day to keep your body hydrated and your blood streaming without a hitch.

Moving Your Body:

• **Normal Activity**: Aim for at least 150 minutes of moderate-power practice or 75 minutes of overwhelming force practice each week. Practice fortifies your heart muscle, further develops blood stream, and oversees weight, all adding to a sound heart.

•   **View as Your Fit:** Pick exercises you appreciate, whether it's energetic strolling, swimming, cycling, moving, or group activities. Consistency is critical, so find a work-out routine you can adhere to long term

•   **Strength Preparing:** Don't disregard strength training! Building muscle mass helps regulate blood pressure and improves on overall cardiovascular health.

Subduing the Pressure Beast:

•   Persistent pressure is a significant risk factor for coronary illness. Practice pressure management procedures like yoga, reflection, profound breathing activities, or investing energy in nature to really oversee pressure.

•   Quality Rest: Aim for long periods of value rest every evening. Lack of sleep can add to hypertension and other heart wellbeing chances. Make a loosening up sleep time routine and lay out a steady rest plan.

Developing Internal Harmony:

• **Mind-Body Connection**: The brain and body are profoundly connected. Rehearses like care reflection can promote emotional wellbeing and lower feelings of anxiety, decidedly influencing your heart wellbeing.

• **Positive Connections**: Encircle yourself with strong and positive individuals. Solid social associations can decrease pressure and give a feeling of having a place, which is valuable for your heart.

• **Laughter is a pain reliever with no side effects**: Giggling is a characteristic pressure reliever. Set aside a few minutes for exercises that give you pleasure and giggling, as it can emphatically affect your heart wellbeing.

Carrying on with a Healthy lifestyle:

• **Limit Liquor Utilization**: Inordinate liquor utilization can raise pulse and increase your risk of coronary illness. Practice control or keep away from liquor through and through if fundamental.

• **Try not to Smoke**: Smoking is a significant risk factor for coronary illness. Stopping smoking is the absolute most significant thing you can accomplish for your heart wellbeing. Look for help if necessary to move beyond the vice.

•   **Normal Exams:** Schedule customary tests with your primary care physician to screen your heart wellbeing. Early recognition and treatment of potential issues are critical for forestalling confusions.

Keep in mind: An all encompassing way to deal with heart wellbeing is a deep rooted venture. By integrating these techniques into your day to day daily schedule, you can make an establishment for a solid, sound heart and a day to day existence loaded up with essentials.

By embracing an all encompassing way to deal with heart wellbeing, you can engage yourself to assume responsibility for your wellbeing and sustain your heart for a long and sound life.

Conclusion

Your Heart - A Lifelong Journey

Your heart is a remarkable organ, tirelessly working to sustain your life. Taking care of it is not just about avoiding disease; it's about embracing a lifestyle that fosters vitality and well-being. The good news is that you have the power to significantly impact your heart health through your choices.

By adopting a holistic approach, you can create a symphony of healthy habits. Nourish your body with nutrient-rich foods, move it with regular exercise, and tame the stress monster with relaxation techniques. Cultivate inner peace through mindfulness and positive relationships, and don't forget the power of laughter!

Remember, a healthy heart is not just about the physical; it's about nurturing your mind, body, and spirit. Schedule regular checkups with your doctor, listen to your body's signals, and don't hesitate to seek professional guidance.

Embrace this journey of self-care. With dedication and a commitment to a healthy lifestyle, you can empower your heart to thrive and live a life filled with joy, purpose, and vibrant health.

Acknowledgement

I wish to thank Almighty God for the inspiration to undertake this project and contribute to the society positively.

About the Author

Leo Chambers is a creative writer and Digital Content Creator.

www.ingramcontent.com/pod-product-compliance
Lightning Source LLC
Chambersburg PA
CBHW050746250726
48653CB00028B/1789